Order this book from :

PRITCHETT & HULL ASSOCIATES, INC.
3440 OAKCLIFF RD NE STE 110
ATLANTA GA 30340-3006

or call toll free: 800-241-4925

This book is only to help you
learn, and should not be used to
replace any of your doctor's advice
or treatment.

Published and distributed by:
Pritchett & Hull Associates, Inc.

Printed in the U.S.A.

How You Can Prevent

Pressure Ulcers

a guide for patients
and family care givers

by Judith L. McKrell

What are pressure ulcers?

Pressure ulcers* are injuries to your skin and the tissue below it. Most often, they happen over bony areas that receive too much pressure or other stress. Pressure squeezes shut blood vessels that take food and oxygen to the skin. If these vessels stay shut for too long, the skin starts to die, and a pressure ulcer forms.

Pressure ulcers are like forest fires. They start small but can quickly become worse and have serious results. But, like forest fires, most pressure ulcers can be prevented.

Follow your doctor or nurse's instructions and the advice in this booklet to lower your risk of pressure ulcers. You will be healthier, more active and find it easier to enjoy life.

This book is only to help you learn. It should not be used to replace any advice or treatment from your nurse, doctor or therapist.

Dear Reader,

Pressure ulcers are no fun! I know because I've had them. That's why writing this book was important to me. I hope it helps you avoid the pain and problems pressure ulcers can bring.

– Judith McKrell

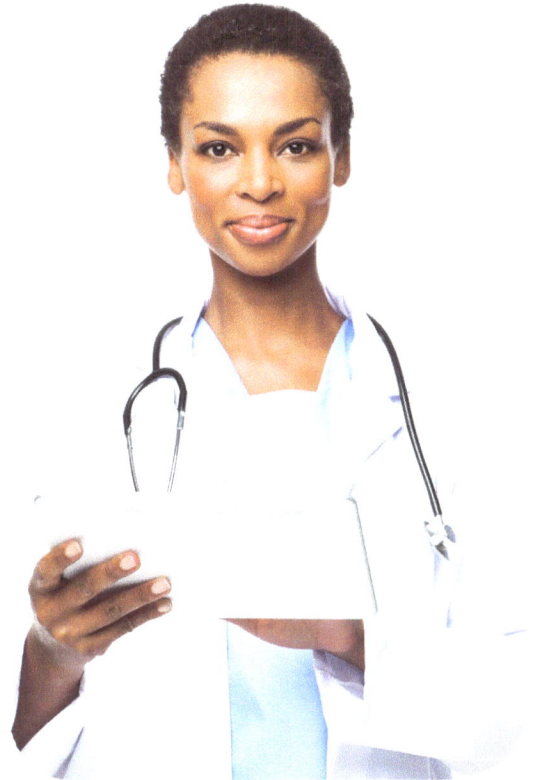

*Other names for pressure ulcer are decubitus ulcer, bedsore and pressure sore.

Why worry about pressure ulcers?

Pressure ulcers can:

- hurt

- cause serious infections that could threaten your life

- disrupt your normal activities for weeks or months while they heal

- be costly and take a lot of time to care for

What causes pressure ulcers?

Pressure

Pressure is the main cause. It can result from:

- lying or sitting too long in one position

- lying or sitting on wrinkled sheets or clothes

- lying or sitting on drainage devices (cath tubing, IV tubing, clamps, etc)

- sitting or lying on small objects left in the bed or chair

Pressure ulcers can start after as little as two hours of pressure.

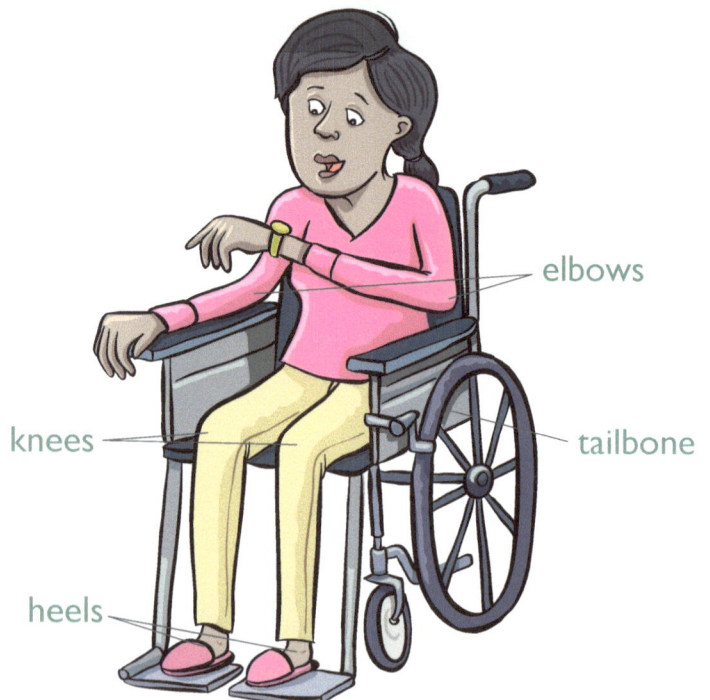

elbows

knees

tailbone

heels

What increases the risk of pressure ulcers?

Shearing and friction

Shearing and friction both happen when your body slides. In shearing, skin pulls away (shears) from the tissue under it, stretching and tearing blood vessels. This reduces the flow of oxygen to the skin.

Friction rubs off the top layer of skin. Shearing and friction can be caused by:

- sliding up or down in the bed or chair

- being dragged rather than lifted

- spasms

- tight clothes and clothes with rough seams or zippers

- restless movement

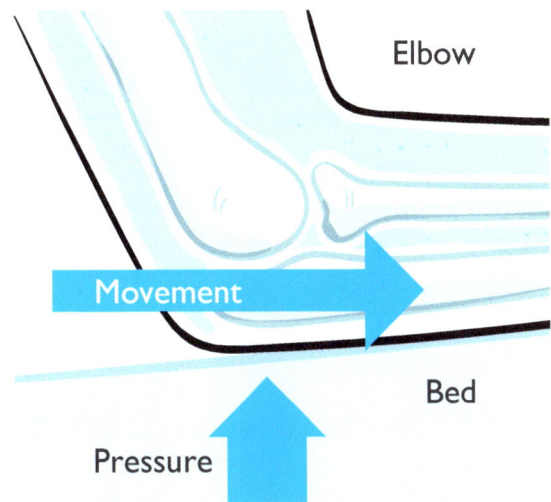

Moisture

Skin can also be irritated by:

- sweat

- urine

- stool (bowel movement)

- moisture left in skin folds

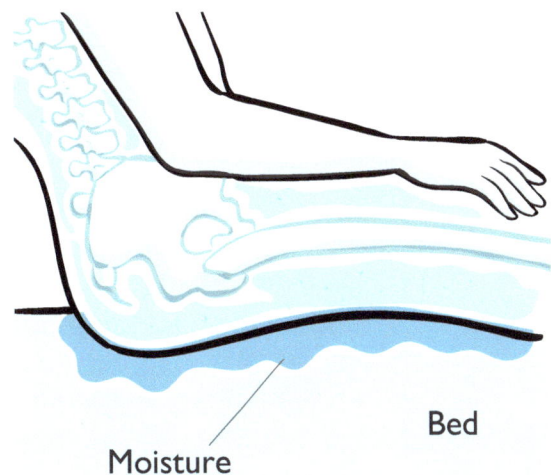

Poor diet

Not eating well can increase your risk for pressure ulcers.
A poor diet can lead to:

- being overweight

- being underweight

- dehydration (not enough fluids)

- anemia (causes slower healing)

You need to eat a well balanced diet with enough protein, calories and vitamins. You also need to drink enough fluids to keep your skin healthy. Ask your doctor or nurse what the right amounts and the best foods are for you.

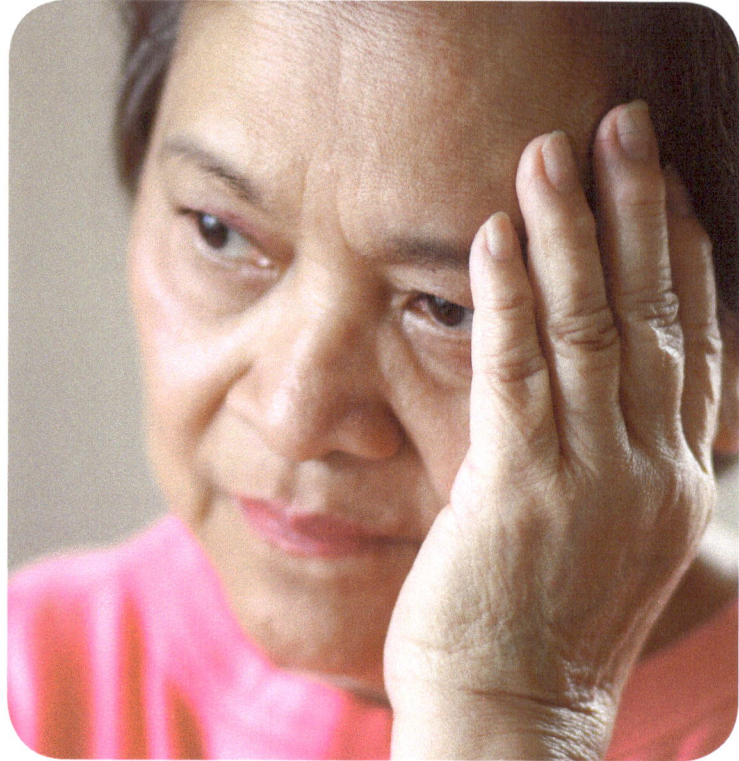

Other factors

Other things that can increase the risk of pressure ulcers are:

- paralysis (can't move, can't feel pain)

- not being mentally alert (not aware of pain)

- aging skin (less elastic)

- diabetes (decreased blood flow)

- hardening of the arteries (less oxygen to tissue)

- swelling (makes tissue stretch so blood supply is not enough)

- smoking (less oxygen to tissue)

How will I know if I'm getting a pressure ulcer?

Check your skin

To find warning signs of a pressure ulcer, you need to check your skin often. You should do this at least once a day and more often if you have a high risk of getting pressure ulcers.

Keep a record of warning signs (see p. 8). This will help you keep track of an ulcer's progress. It will also tell your doctor or nurse what he or she needs to know to prescribe treatment.

Checking may seem like a lot of bother at first, but once you know what, how and where to look, it will become routine. Remember: a little checking time now beats a lot of healing time later.

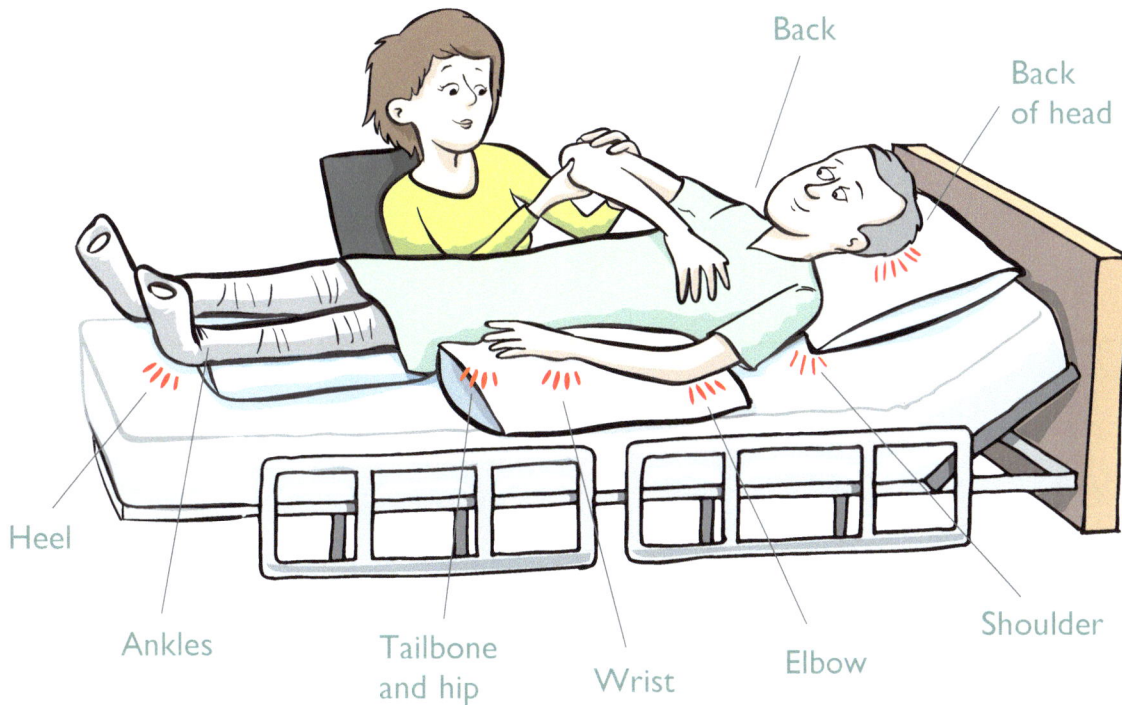

Back

Back of head

Heel

Ankles

Tailbone and hip

Wrist

Elbow

Shoulder

When checking your skin, look at all of the bony and other areas shown below. As you turn and move throughout the day, check all skin areas getting pressure, friction or moisture. Carefully check areas where you can feel bone near the skin or where the bone sticks up. Some of these places are near the tailbone, hip, ankles and heels.

Check all areas that you can see, then use a mirror to check those you cannot. Touch the areas to see if they feel warm or hard. If you cannot stand, you will need to do this in bed. If you cannot turn, feel or hold a mirror yourself, you will need someone to help you.

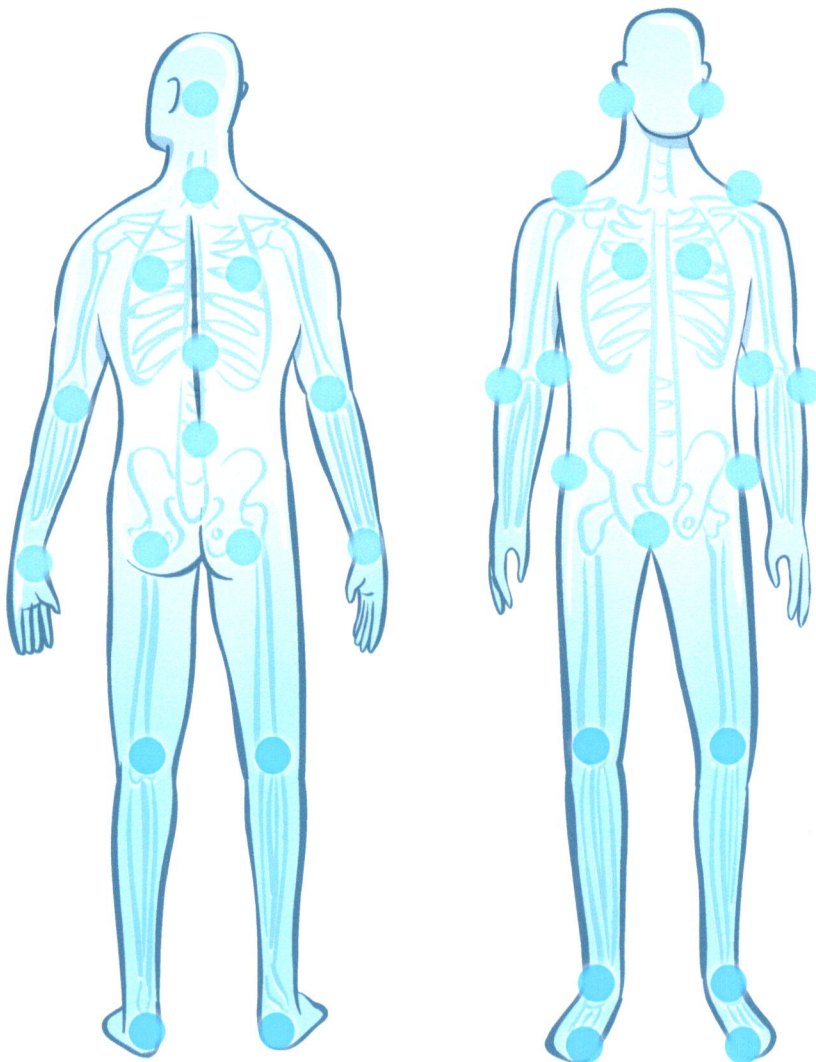

Warning signs to look for

- in light-skinned people, pink or red colored areas that do not turn white when touched; in dark-skinned people, blue or purple areas

- areas that feel hard and/or warm

- blisters, scrapes or other broken skin

- swelling

- pain over bony area

Record problem signs and areas on the chart in the back of this book.

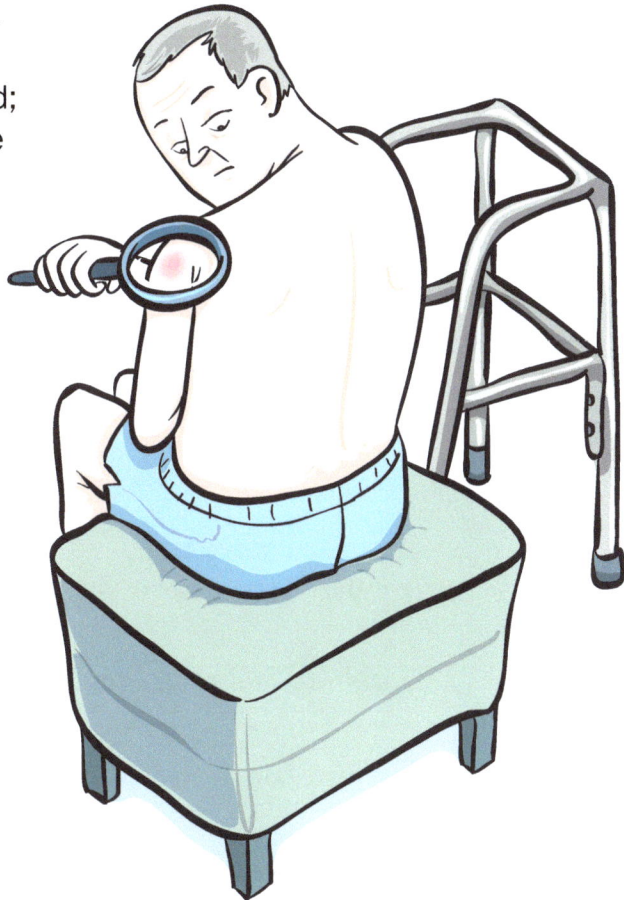

What to do about warning signs

If you find a pressure ulcer, try to figure out what caused it. Avoid shear and friction. Keep skin clean and dry. Stay off of the area. Get rid of the pressure!

Remove pressure from red or purple areas and check them often. If they last more than 30 minutes to an hour, it could mean deep tissue damage. If they do not go away within a few hours, call your doctor or nurse. Report any areas with broken skin at once.

Your risk factors

In the list below, check the risk factors that apply to you. The more you check, the greater your risk of pressure ulcers. But, even a high risk does not mean you're doomed. It simply means you must be extra careful to follow steps to prevent them. **You can prevent most pressure ulcers!**

Risk Factors

In bed or wheelchair most of time

Unable to move self
(paralyzed, comatose, broken hip, etc.)

Unable to feel pressure or pain

Spasms; slide in bed or chair often

Cannot control bladder or bowels

Sweat a lot

Not mentally alert (not aware of pressure or pain or how to prevent it)

Poor diet, over- or underweight, dehydrated

Aging skin

Diabetes, anemia, poor blood flow to the arteries, swelling or other factors such as smoking

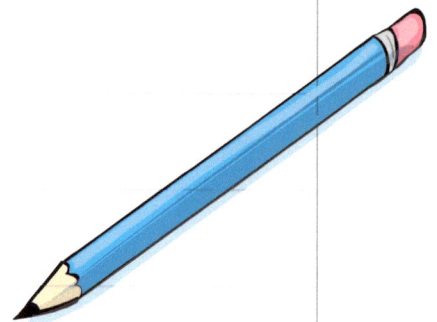

How can I prevent pressure ulcers?

Change positions often

Here are some general rules for positioning. Ask your doctor or nurse what is best for you.

In bed

1. Shift your weight at least every hour. Change positions at least every two hours. Make sure your weight is spread evenly with no pressure on bony areas.

Lying on side

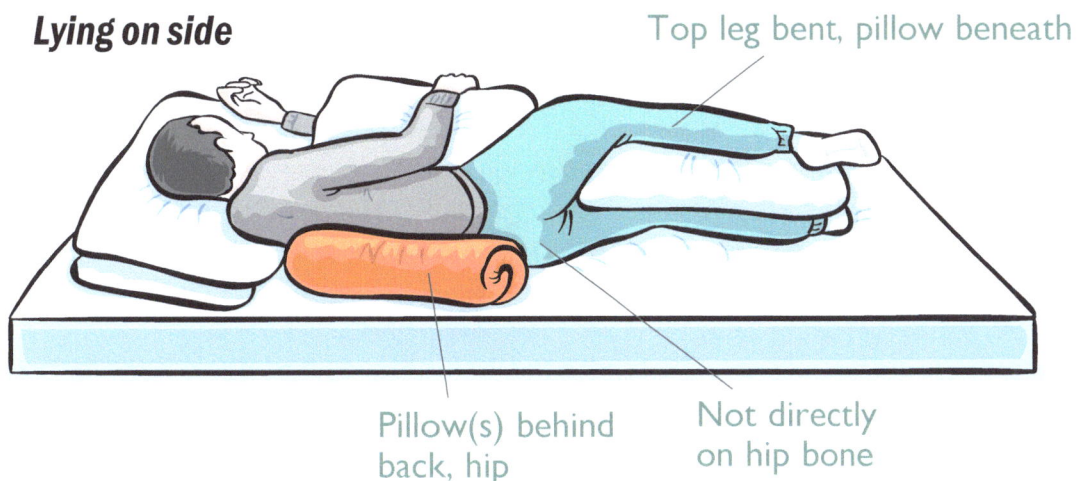

Top leg bent, pillow beneath

Pillow(s) behind back, hip

Not directly on hip bone

Lying on back

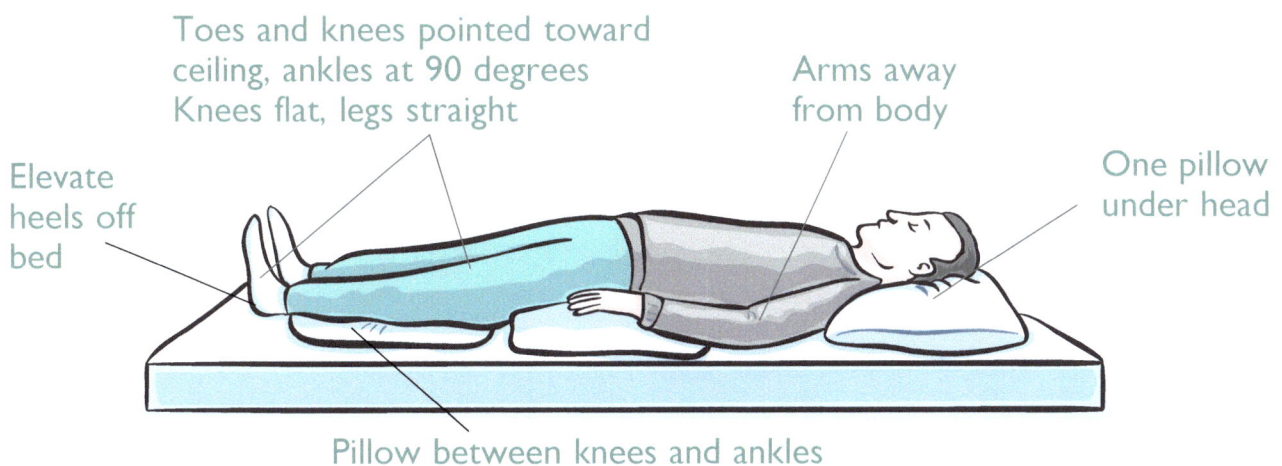

Toes and knees pointed toward ceiling, ankles at 90 degrees
Knees flat, legs straight

Arms away from body

One pillow under head

Elevate heels off bed

Pillow between knees and ankles

Lying on stomach

This position lets you sleep through the night without having to turn as often. The pillows help to reduce pressure.

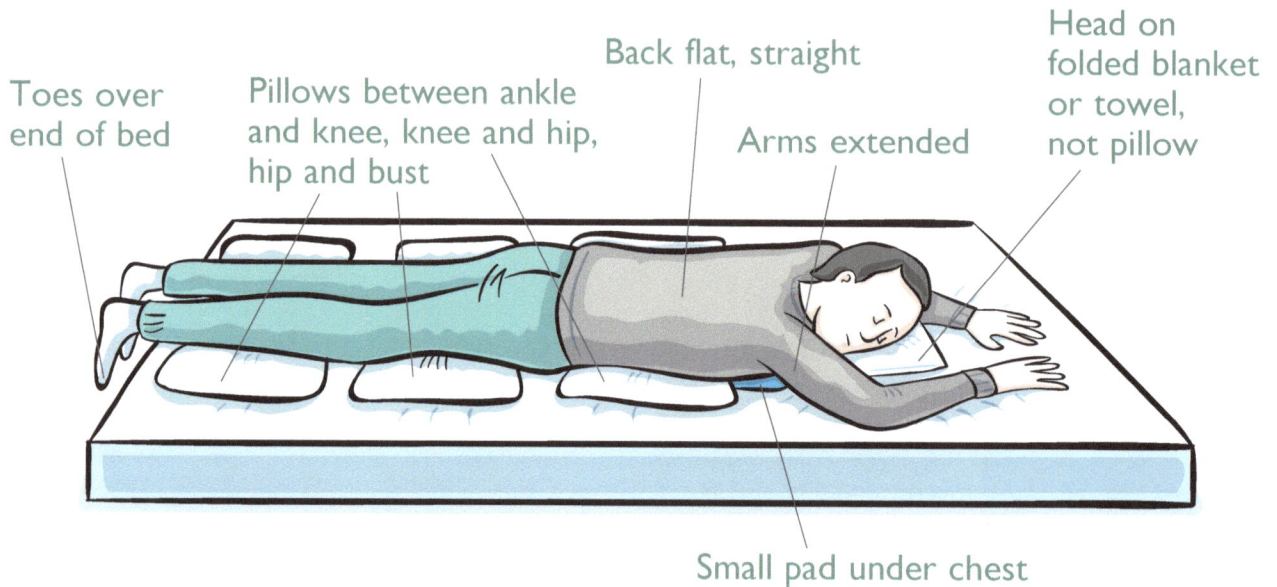

Toes over end of bed

Pillows between ankle and knee, knee and hip, hip and bust

Back flat, straight

Arms extended

Head on folded blanket or towel, not pillow

Small pad under chest

2. Keep track of when you turn. This is even more important if you depend on others to turn you. Set a timer or make a turning "clock," like the one on page 20. Or, keep a notebook, writing down each time you turn, what position you turn to and if there are any marks on your skin that need to be watched.

3. Work your turning schedule around your activities. For example, schedule lying on your back for mealtimes.

If you cannot care for yourself, teach your care givers how to prevent pressure ulcers.

If you are a care giver, work with the person to prevent ulcers. If the person is not mentally alert, you will need to take responsibility for the prevention of pressure ulcers.

In a chair or wheelchair

1. Maintain good posture. Do not slump.

2. Shift your weight at least every 15 minutes. To do this, try one of these:

- Lift your hips as you lean from side to side.

- With your safety belt on, put your feet flat on the floor. Lean forward and lift your weight from the chair.

- Press down on the arms of the chair and lift your weight off the seat.

- Have someone sit behind you and tilt your chair back. The wheelchair handles should rest on the person's lap. Use a pillow for your head.

3. Change positions at least every hour.

4. Be careful to avoid scrapes, bumps and bruises when switching between the bed and chair.

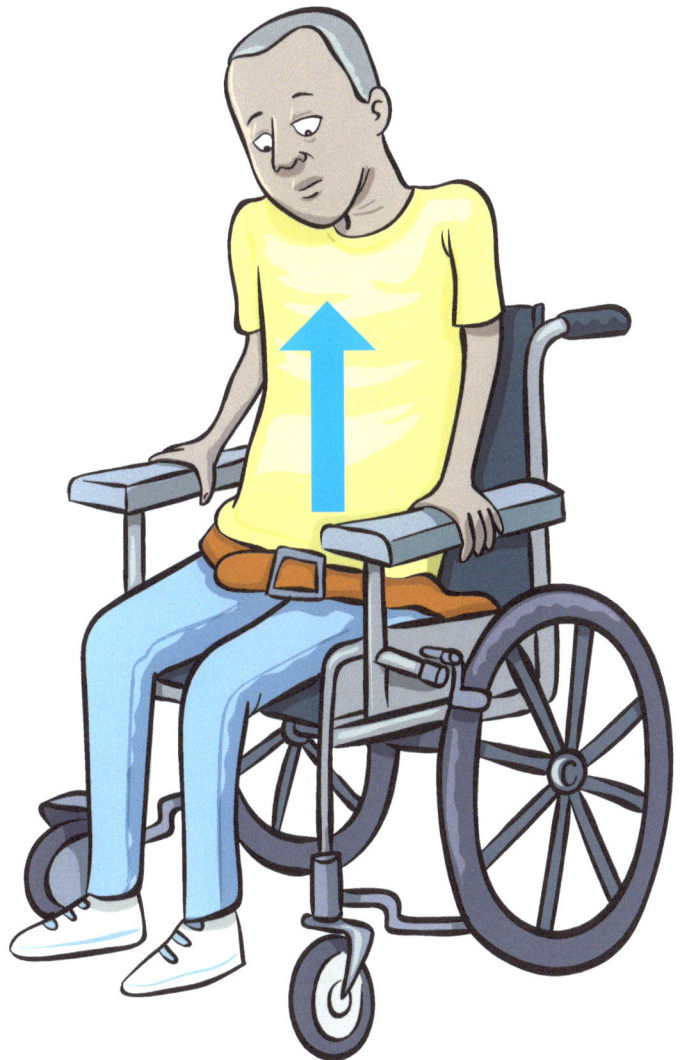

CAUTION

Always lock your wheelchair before shifting weight.

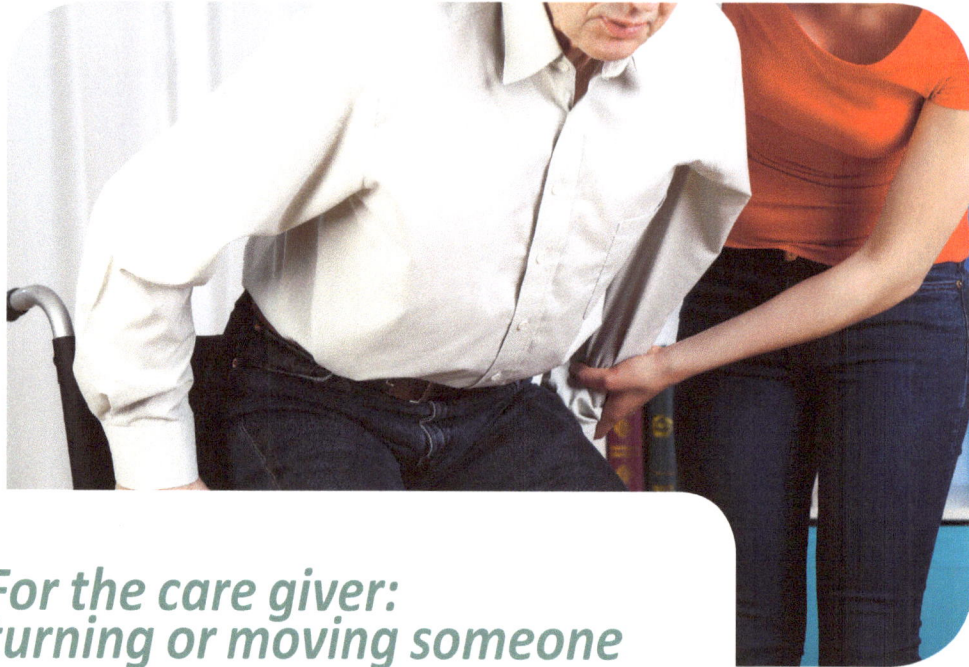

For the care giver: turning or moving someone

1. Ask the doctor or nurse to show you how. Practice while she watches.

2. When you turn or move someone:

- Bend your hips and knees, keeping your back straight. Use your legs to lift, not your back.

- Keep your feet apart with one foot in front of the other.

- Use safety devices such as bed rails and wheelchair locks.

- When moving, hold the person close to your body. Support his body with yours.

- Lift or roll, don't slide the person.

- Always turn the person toward you.

- Make sure he is comfortable, with no pressure on bony areas.

Use pressure relief devices

Before you buy or use a device, ask your doctor or nurse which is best for you. Also, check with your insurance company to see if it is covered. Find out where devices can be bought or rented, and shop around to get the best price.

In bed

1. To help **spread your weight evenly**, use a gel, water, air, foam or other special mattress.

2. To keep your knees from touching, place a pillow or wedge between them. Do the same for your ankles. Use other pillows or wedges as needed for propping. But, **don't use a back wedge.** This shifts weight to the bony part of your back.

3. **Wear foam or gel heel protectors.** Or, place a pillow under your legs between your ankles and calves to keep your heels off the bed. Never put a pillow under just your knees. This could cut off blood flow.

4. To keep your feet at 90 degrees, use a padded footboard. If feeling and blood supply are good, you can wear thick sports socks and loosely tied high top tennis shoes for 2 to 3 hours at a time.

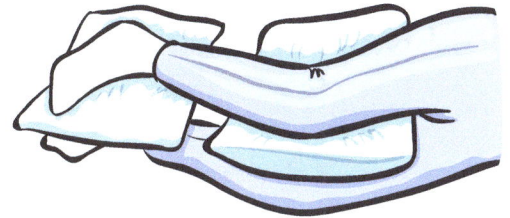

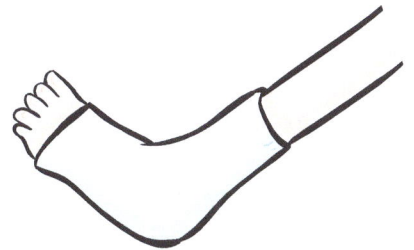

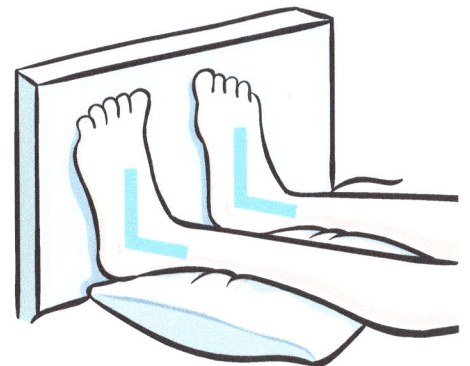

⚠ CAUTION

Don't use donut-type cushions. They can cut off blood flow.

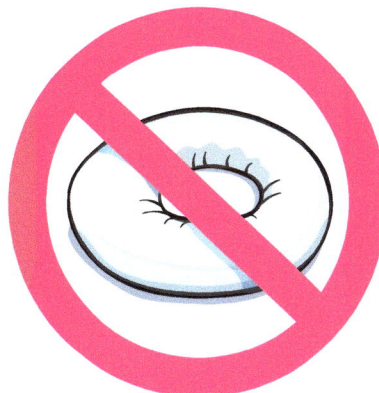

5. To keep sheets and blankets from resting on your legs and feet, try using a bed cradle. (It is like a tent.)

6. For lifting, a drawsheet can be used by 2 care givers. A trapeze or mechanical lift may be helpful if there is only 1 care giver.

In a chair or wheelchair

1. To relieve pressure, use a foam, air, gel or other special cushion.

2. Do not use a donut-type cushion. It can reduce blood flow, increasing the chance of pressure sores.

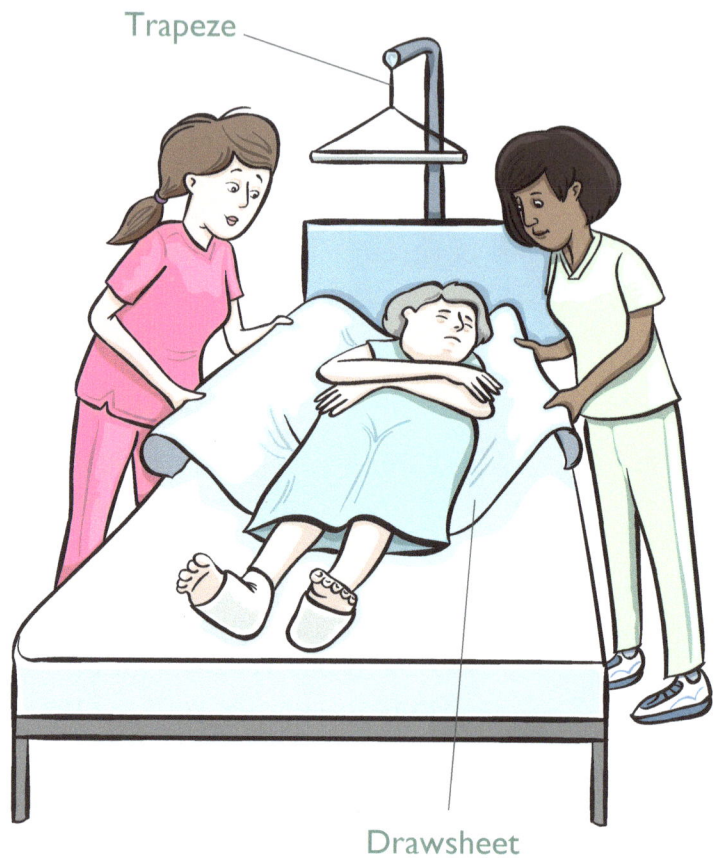

Trapeze

Drawsheet

Move as much as you can

1. Stay out of bed as much as you are allowed. Moving around makes blood flow better and helps your skin stay healthy.

2. If you can, walk or do other exercise to keep up good blood flow. Ask your doctor or nurse about range of motion exercises and physical therapy.

3. Change chairs once in a while. Any activity will help you change position and prevent pressure ulcers.

Avoid shearing and friction

1. Except for eating, don't raise the head of the bed higher than 30 degrees. This prevents sliding. The best position is mostly flat or semi-flat (15 degrees). Raising the foot of the bed slightly will also help prevent sliding.

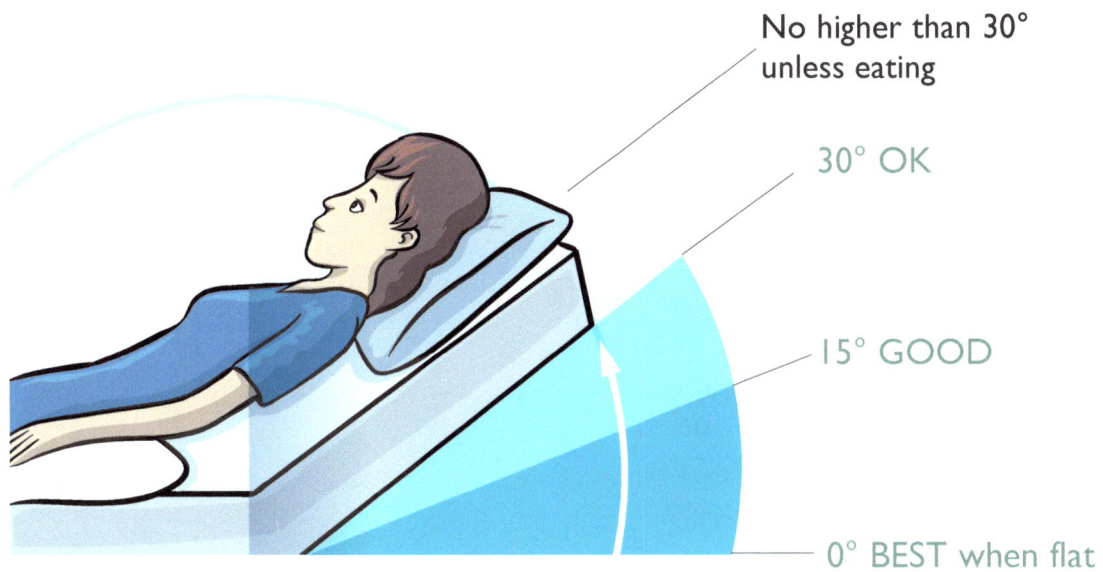

No higher than 30° unless eating

30° OK

15° GOOD

0° BEST when flat

2. Lift, don't slide, when moving in or between the bed and chair. If needed, use a drawsheet or mechanical lifting device.

3. If restless movement or spasms are a problem, talk to your doctor about how to get relief.

4. Avoid tight or rough clothing and those with thick seams or folds, such as jeans. Clothing that is too loose can bunch up and form wrinkles that put pressure on the skin.

5. Use padding or protective dressings on bony areas, like knees and elbows.

6. Dry skin is less elastic and easier to damage. Use cream or oil to keep your skin from getting too dry. Rub it in well, so it doesn't leave your skin too moist.

Keep clean, stay dry

1. Bathe or shower regularly. Use warm (not hot) water, a mild soap and a soft cloth.

2. Pat skin dry. Don't rub. Be sure to dry skin folds.

3. Use cream or lotion to prevent dry skin. Avoid dry or cold air—this will dry skin.

4. Do not massage over bony areas that are red or purple. This is the first sign of pressure and should be reported to your doctor or nurse.

5. When bowel or bladder control is a problem, clean skin as soon as it is soiled. Change wet sheets and clothes at once.

6. Use pads or briefs that pull moisture away from the skin. Use a single layer of padding. Multiple layers can wrinkle and cause sweating.

7. Use an ointment or cream to protect skin from urine or stool.

8. Make sure drainage devices, such as tubes, are not under your body.

9. Don't sit on a toilet or bedpan for long periods of time. This can restrict blood flow and cause pressure ulcers.

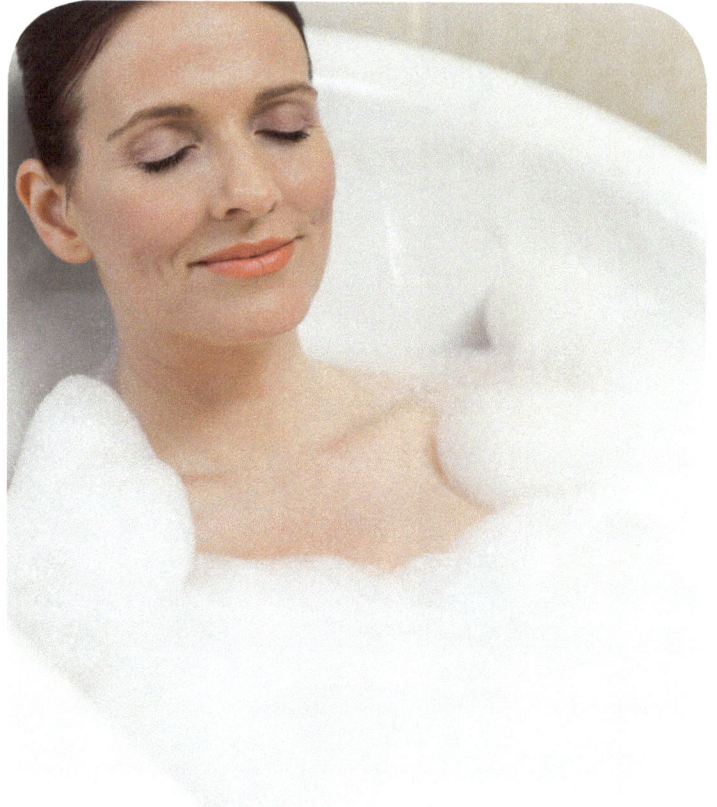

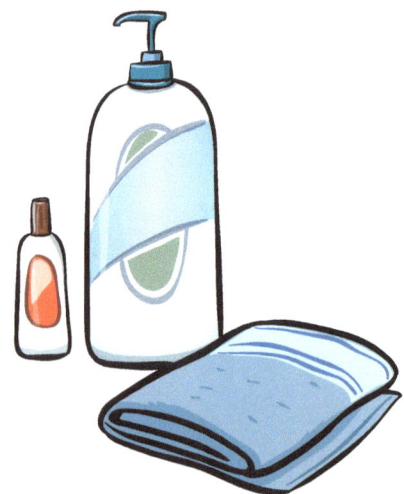

Eat a healthy diet

1. Eat a balanced diet. Foods high in protein, iron, zinc, Vitamin A, Vitamin C and B vitamins promote healthy skin.

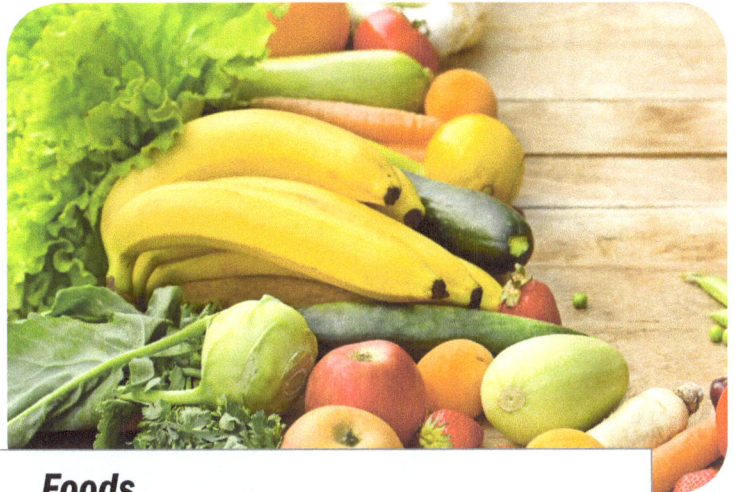

Foods

Protein	meats, poultry, eggs, fish, tofu, dairy products, whole grain breads and cereals, dried peas, beans or nuts
Iron	liver, meats, oysters, whole grain breads and cereals, dried fruits, nuts, dark green leafy vegetables
Zinc	beans and lentils, meats, oysters, eggs, whole grain breads and cereals
Vitamin A	liver, carrots, cantaloupe, sweet potatoes, spinach, broccoli, other yellow and dark green fruits and vegetables
Vitamin C	citrus fruits, strawberries, cantaloupe, tomatoes, sweet peppers, sweet potatoes, cabbage, broccoli, dark green leafy vegetables
B Vitamins	meats, poultry, fish, eggs, dairy foods, whole grain breads and cereals, dried beans and peas, dark green leafy vegetables

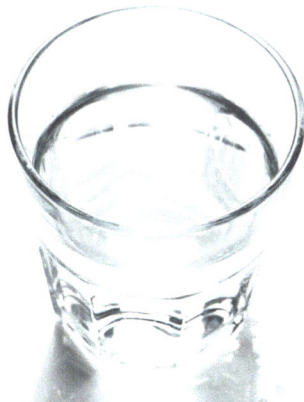

2. If you cannot eat a normal diet, talk to your doctor or nurse about diet supplements. If you are over- or underweight, ask about a special diet.

3. Unless your fluids are restricted, drink plenty of water, at least a liter (about 4 – 8oz glasses) a day. Drink more water if you can.

Other tips to prevent pressure ulcers

1. After you turn or move, check to see that there are no wrinkles in sheets or clothes. Keep track of small objects such as combs, nail files, drainage caps, crumbs, etc. Sitting or lying on any of these can cause pressure ulcers.

2. Be careful with cigarettes, hot drinks and the temperature of tub and shower water. Don't use hot water bottles or other heating devices on parts of your body that have little or no feeling.

3. If swelling is a problem, elevate your hands and feet. Wear support hose if your doctor or nurse recommends them. Be sure you remove the hose on a regular schedule.

4. If you will be having anesthesia or taking medicine that will cause you to be less alert, write down instructions about your skin care for others to follow.

5. Older adults and people with paralysis (can't feel), anemia, diabetes or poor blood flow should pay special attention to their skin.

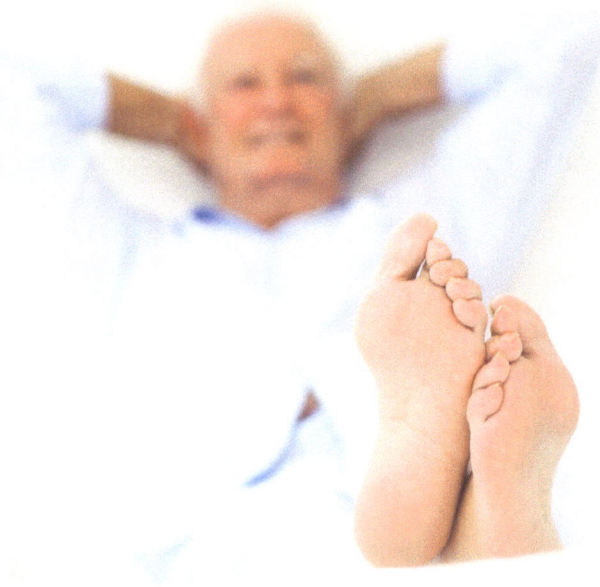

My plan for preventing pressure ulcers

Talk with your doctor or nurse about the best plan for you.

Change positions often

In bed

Fill in the position you should be turned to at each time.
Plan your turning schedule around your activities.

midnight   noon

12   2am   12   2pm
10am   10pm
8am   4am   8pm   4pm
6am   6pm

In chair

Shift weight every_____

Method(s) to use _____

_____

Change positions every_____

Pritchett & Hull Associates, Inc., Atlanta, GA
Patients and their families may copy this page.

Use pressure relief devices

Device	Special Instructions

Move as much as possible

Activities	How Often

Avoid shearing and friction

Lifting methods to use_____

_____

How much to raise head of bed (see p. 16)_____

Other_____

_____

_____

Pritchett & Hull Associates, Inc., Atlanta, GA
Patients and their families may copy this page.

21

Keep clean, stay dry

Bathe (how often)_____

Soaps, ointments, creams to use_____

Other_____

Eat a healthy diet

Foods	How Much	How Often

Amount of fluids to drink_____

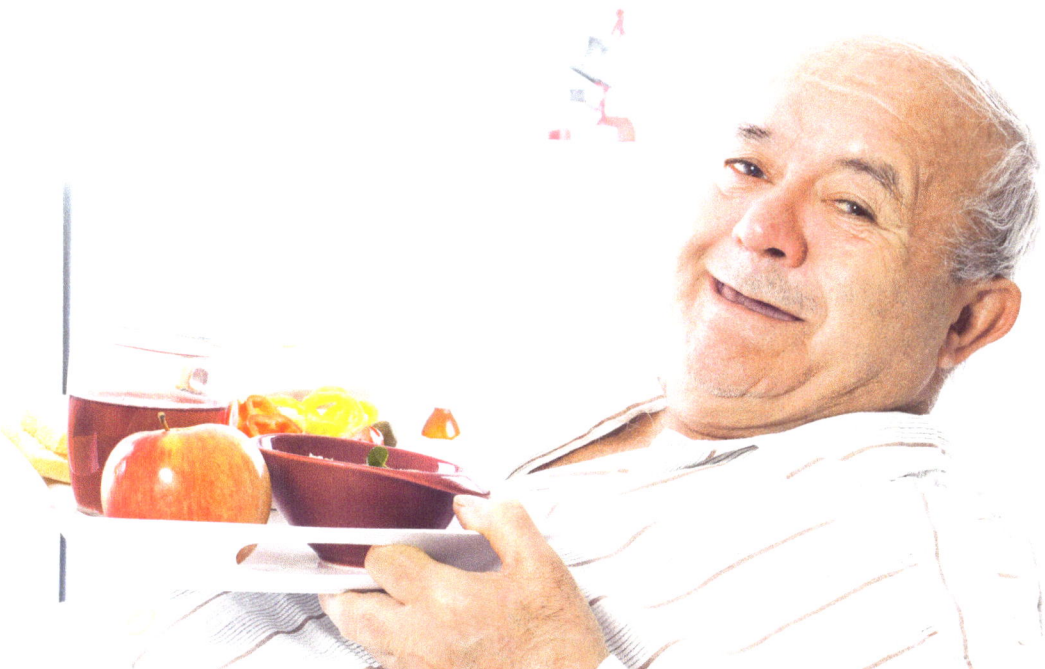

Pritchett & Hull Associates, Inc., Atlanta, GA
Patients and their families may copy this page.

Check skin

Copy this page, then use it as the start of an ongoing record.

How often to check:

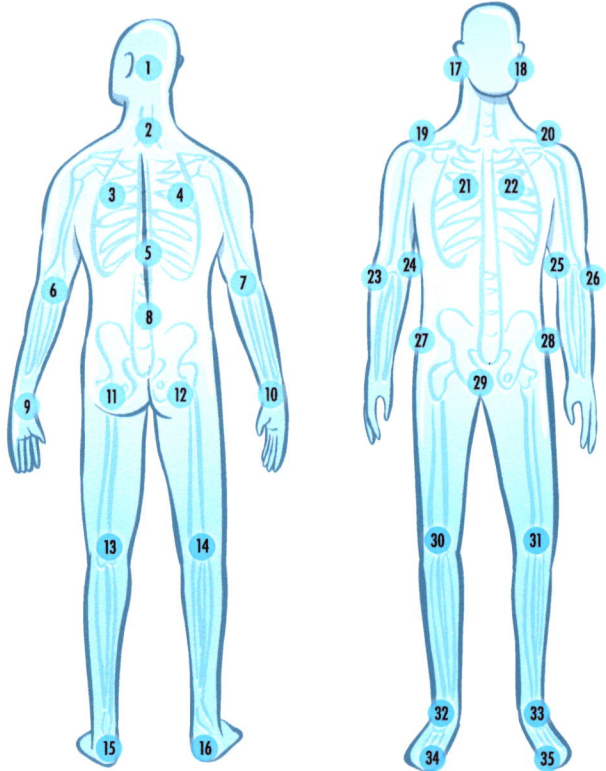

_____

Date	Time	# of Problem Area	How It Looks

Pritchett & Hull Associates, Inc., Atlanta, GA
Patients and their families may copy this page.

23

For more information

Phone numbers

Doctor: _____

Nurse: _____

Other: _____

For information for patients, care givers and families
at home, contact:

National Pressure Ulcer Advisory Panel
Ste 500 East
1025 Thomas Jefferson St NW
Washington, DC 20007
(202)-521-6789
www.npuap.org

To find a wound care nurse in your area, contact:

Wound, Ostomy and Continence Nurses Society
1120 Route 73 Ste 200
Mount Laurel NJ 08054
(888)-224-9626
www.wocn.org

Notes

www.ingramcontent.com/pod-product-compliance
Lightning Source LLC
Chambersburg PA
CBHW060857270326
41934CB00003B/183